THE PMHNP CLINICAL HANDBOOK

Practical Psychiatry for Everyday Practice

Advanced Practice Series — Volume 2

Liberty Olive RB Macias, DNP, APRN, PMHNP-BC

Advanced Practice

PROFESSIONAL DISCLAIMER

This publication is intended for educational and professional development purposes only. It is not intended to replace independent clinical judgment, comprehensive clinical references, current prescribing information, applicable clinical guidelines, consultation, supervision, or individualized patient assessment and treatment.

Clinical information, recommendations, medications, regulations, and standards of practice may change over time. Readers are responsible for verifying current information and practicing in accordance with their professional scope, applicable laws and regulations, organizational policies, professional standards, and the circumstances of each individual patient.

The clinical examples, frameworks, checklists, and other materials presented in this handbook are illustrative and should not be interpreted as establishing a standard of care or as requiring a particular clinical decision, treatment, or course of action.

The author and publisher assume no responsibility for clinical decisions or outcomes resulting from the use or interpretation of information contained in this publication.

DEDICATION

To Dr. Mubashir Farooqi

For your mentorship, encouragement, and unwavering support—not only of my professional journey, but of my entrepreneurial pursuits and the many ideas I dared to chase. Thank you for opening doors, expanding my world through the people and opportunities you introduced me to, and believing in possibilities I was still learning to see.

And most of all, thank you for encouraging me to fly while always knowing when to pull me gently back to earth.

CONTENTS

PREFACE

From Knowing Psychiatry to Practicing It

Graduate education gives us the foundation for psychiatric practice. We learn assessment, diagnosis, psychopharmacology, treatment planning, ethics, and the principles that guide safe patient care.

Then we begin practicing and we discover that knowing psychiatry and practicing psychiatry are not quite the same thing.

Real patients rarely arrive organized according to diagnostic criteria. Their histories may be incomplete. Symptoms overlap. Medications that should work sometimes do not. Treatments that worked before may no longer work. Laboratory results, medical conditions, family concerns, insurance limitations, patient preferences, and competing priorities all become part of a decision that still has to be made.

The PMHNP Clinical Handbook was created for those moments.

This handbook is not intended to replace comprehensive psychiatric textbooks, prescribing references, current clinical guidelines, or your own professional judgment. It is a practical companion designed to help bridge what we learn in training with what we encounter in everyday psychiatric practice.

This handbook is intended not simply to provide answers, but to help you develop a way of thinking through the questions that psychiatric practice repeatedly presents.

You will not always know the answer immediately. Clinical confidence does not come from knowing everything. It develops from learning how to recognize what matters, what you still need to know, when to seek consultation, and how to make thoughtful decisions with the information available to you.

My hope is that this handbook becomes the kind of resource you return to—not because it contains everything you need to know about psychiatry, but because it helps you find your footing when clinical practice becomes complicated.

Use it as a guide. Question it when appropriate. Continue learning. And let experience refine what no handbook can fully teach.

Liberty Olive RB Macias, DNP, APRN, PMHNP-BC

Welcome to *The PMHNP Clinical Handbook.*

If *The New PMHNP* was written to prepare you mentally and professionally for your transition into practice, this handbook was written to help you navigate the realities of clinical practice.

This is not intended to replace your graduate education, board review materials, clinical guidelines, or supervising physicians and mentors.

Instead, it serves as a practical companion—a resource you can return to when you need guidance on the everyday challenges of psychiatric practice.

The chapters are organized in the same sequence that many clinicians experience during their first year:

- Preparing for practice
- Evaluating patients
- Developing differential diagnoses
- Creating treatment plans
- Prescribing medications safely
- Documenting effectively
- Managing difficult situations
- Building a sustainable career

Throughout the book, you will find several recurring features designed to reinforce learning and encourage clinical reasoning.

Clinical Pearl

A concise teaching point based on clinical experience that highlights an important concept or practical tip.

Common Misstep

A frequent mistake made by new clinicians, along with strategies to avoid it.

Clinical Reasoning in Action

A real-world patient scenario that demonstrates how experienced clinicians think through assessment, diagnosis, and management.

Liberty's Lesson
Personal reflections drawn from years of clinical practice, teaching, mentorship, and leadership.

Quick Checklist
A practical summary you can review before clinic or while developing your own workflow.

Psychiatry is a profession built on continuous learning. No handbook can give every answer, but it can help you ask better questions, think more critically, and practice more confidently.

I hope this book becomes a trusted companion throughout your career.

Part I

Before Your First Patient

Graduation marks an important milestone but becoming licensed and board certified is only the beginning of your professional journey.

Before you evaluate your first patient, there are several practical steps that will influence your ability to practice safely, efficiently, and successfully.

Understanding licensure, credentialing, malpractice coverage, and employment considerations will help you enter practice with confidence and avoid many of the frustrations experienced by new graduates.

The purpose of this section is to help you build the professional foundation that supports excellent clinical care.

Chapter 1

Now You are a PMHNP…
What Happens Next?

"Graduation marks the end of your formal education—but the beginning of your professional career."

One of the most common questions new graduates ask is, *"What do I do now?"*

After years of coursework, clinical rotations, and board preparation, it is easy to assume that passing your certification examination means you are immediately ready to begin seeing patients. In reality, there are several important administrative and professional steps that must occur before your first day in clinic.

Although these tasks may seem less exciting than diagnosing and treating psychiatric disorders, they are essential components of professional practice. Completing them thoughtfully will make your transition into practice much smoother.

Licensure

Your state Advanced Practice Registered Nurse (APRN) license grants the legal authority to practice according to your state's laws and regulations.

Requirements differ across states, and it is your responsibility to understand the scope of practice where you intend to work.

Keep careful records of license renewal dates, continuing education requirements, and any state-specific prescribing regulations. Developing good organizational habits early in your career will help prevent unnecessary stress later.

Clinical Pearl

Create a professional file containing copies of every license, certification, DEA registration, NPI confirmation, malpractice policy, curriculum vitae, immunization record, and continuing education certificate. You will be surprised how often these documents are requested.

Board Certification

Passing your national certification examination shows that you have met the minimum standards required for entry into practice.

Certification is not the finish line.

Psychiatry continues to evolve rapidly through new research, medications, technologies, and clinical guidelines. Maintaining certification should be viewed as an opportunity to continue growing rather than simply fulfilling a requirement.

DEA Registration

If your practice includes prescribing controlled substances, you will need a DEA registration in addition to your state prescribing authority. Many employers help new graduates with this process, but understanding the requirements yourself is an important professional responsibility.

Become familiar with federal regulations, your state's controlled substance laws, and your organization's prescribing policies before writing your first prescription.

Common Misstep

Waiting until your first day of employment to apply for DEA registration.
DEA processing can take time and may delay your ability to prescribe controlled medications.

National Provider Identifier (NPI)

One of the first administrative tasks after obtaining your APRN license is applying for a **National Provider Identifier (NPI)**. An NPI is a unique 10-digit identification number assigned by the Centers for Medicare & Medicaid Services (CMS) and is used nationwide to identify healthcare providers for billing, credentialing, referrals, and electronic healthcare transactions.

There are two types of NPIs:

Type 1 NPI – Individual Provider

Every PMHNP should obtain a **Type 1 NPI**. This number belongs to you as an individual clinician and remains with you throughout your career, regardless of where you work. If you change employers, relocate to another state, or open your own practice, your Type 1 NPI stays the same.

You will use your Type 1 NPI for:

- Insurance billing
- Electronic prescribing
- Hospital credentialing
- Medicare and Medicaid enrollment
- Referrals and consultations
- Laboratory and imaging orders (when applicable)

Type 2 NPI – Organization

A **Type 2 NPI** is assigned to organizations rather than individuals. Hospitals, clinics, group practices, corporations, and healthcare organizations typically obtain a Type 2 NPI.

If you eventually establish your own professional corporation or private practice, your business may need its own Type 2 NPI while you continue using your personal Type 1 NPI as the treating clinician.

Clinical Pearl

Think of your **Type 1 NPI as your professional identity** and a **Type 2 NPI as your practice's identity**.

Credentialing

Credentialing often surprises new graduates because it is one of the least discussed topics during graduate school. Many new PMHNPs are surprised to learn that obtaining a license and board certification does not automatically allow them to see insured patients.

Before you can provide reimbursable services, healthcare organizations and insurance companies must verify your qualifications through a process called **credentialing**.

This process may include verification of your education, certification, licensure, work history, references, malpractice history, and other professional credentials.

Insurance credentialing frequently takes several months. Whenever possible, begin this process as early as possible after accepting a position.

Clinical Pearl

Credentialing delays are common. Plan financially for the possibility that your first paycheck may arrive later than expected.

Hospital Credentialing

If you plan to work in an inpatient psychiatric unit, emergency department, consultation-liaison service, or any setting requiring hospital privileges, the hospital will conduct its own credentialing process.

Hospital credentialing may include:

- Verification of education and training
- APRN license verification
- National board certification
- DEA registration
- Work history
- Professional references
- Background checks
- Malpractice claims history
- Immunization and occupational health requirements

Hospitals may also grant **clinical privileges**, which define the procedures and services you are authorized to perform within that institution.

Insurance Credentialing

Insurance credentialing allows you to become an **in-network provider** with commercial insurance companies and government healthcare programs.
Each insurance company conducts its own review and may request documentation such as:

- State licenses
- National certification

- DEA registration
- NPI
- Professional liability insurance
- Curriculum vitae
- Practice location information

Until credentialing is complete, many insurance companies will not reimburse for services you provide.

Medicare Enrollment

If you plan to treat Medicare beneficiaries, you must enroll as a Medicare provider through CMS. Many employers assist with this process, but understanding the requirements allows you to monitor your enrollment status and avoid unnecessary delays.

Medicaid Enrollment

Medicaid enrollment is administered at the state level. Each state's Medicaid program has its own application process and documentation requirements. If you practice in multiple states, separate enrollment may be required for each state's Medicaid program.

CAQH

One of the most important resources for credentialing is the **Council for Affordable Quality Healthcare (CAQH)** Provider Data Portal.
Rather than completing separate applications for every insurance company, you enter your professional information into the CAQH database. Participating insurers retrieve your information directly from your CAQH profile during the credentialing process.

Your CAQH profile includes:

- Education
- Licensure
- Certification
- Practice locations
- Work history
- Malpractice coverage
- DEA registration
- Professional references

Your responsibility does not end after creating the profile.

CAQH information must be reviewed, updated, and re-attested regularly to remain current.

Common Misstep

Accepting a position and assuming your employer will manage every aspect of credentialing.

Even when employers assist with the process, you remain responsible for submitting requested documents promptly, monitoring application status, and keeping your credentials current.

Malpractice Insurance

Professional liability insurance is one of the most important safeguards in your career.

Although many employers provide malpractice coverage, every PMHNP should understand the type of policy they are covered under and what protections it offers.

Ask questions such as:

- *Is the policy occurrence-based or claims-made?*
- *Is tail coverage included?*
- *Are telepsychiatry services covered?*
- *Does the policy extend to volunteer activities or moonlighting?*

Understanding your coverage is part of practicing responsibly.

Occurrence Policy

An **occurrence policy** covers claims arising from incidents that occurred while the policy was active, even if the lawsuit is filed years later.
Once the policy period has passed, you remain protected for events that occurred during that time.

Occurrence policies are more expensive but provide long-term peace of mind.

Claims-Made Policy

A **claims-made policy** provides coverage only if **both** the clinical event and the legal claim occur while the policy is active.

If you leave your employer or allow the policy to expire, future claims related to your previous practice may not be covered unless additional protection is obtained.

Tail Coverage

Tail coverage extends protection after a claims-made policy ends.
If you leave an employer with claims-made coverage, determine:

- *Who is responsible for purchasing tail coverage?*
- *Is it included in your employment contract?*
- *What are the costs?*

These questions should be answered before accepting a position—not after resigning.

Employer Coverage

Never assume your employer's malpractice policy covers every aspect of your practice.

Ask questions such as:

- *Does coverage include telepsychiatry?*
- *Are moonlighting activities covered?*
- *Does coverage extend to volunteer work?*
- *Are supervising responsibilities included?*
- *Are legal defense costs covered?*

Request a copy of the policy summary and understand its limitations.

Liberty's Lesson

One of the best pieces of professional advice I received early in my career was simple: **understand the business side of practice.**

Most graduate programs teach us how to diagnose psychiatric disorders, prescribe medications, and provide compassionate care. Few teach us about credentialing, liability insurance, contracts, or reimbursement.

Learning these topics will not make you less of a clinician—it will make you a more informed professional. The more you understand how healthcare systems work, the better prepared you will be to make decisions that protect both your patients and your career.

Finding Your First Job

Perhaps the most important career decision you will make as a new PMHNP is choosing your first employer.

Many graduates focus primarily on salary.

While compensation is certainly important, your first position should also provide mentorship, reasonable patient volumes, structured orientation, opportunities for consultation, and a supportive learning environment.

The quality of your first year may influence your confidence and professional development for years to come.

Liberty's Lesson

Choose your first job for the person you will become—not simply for the salary you will earn.

A workplace that encourages questions, values collaboration, and invests in your professional growth will often provide far greater long-term rewards than one that offers a higher paycheck but little support.

Clinical Reasoning in Action

"Can I Start Seeing Patients Tomorrow?"

A newly certified PMHNP accepts an outpatient psychiatry position and is eager to begin. During orientation, they learn that their insurance credentialing has not yet been completed. Although they can observe patient visits and participate in training, they cannot independently bill for clinical services.

Rather than viewing this delay as a setback, they use the time to learn the electronic health record, review clinic workflows, become familiar with documentation expectations, observe experienced clinicians, and build relationships with new colleagues.

By the time credentialing is complete, they feel far more prepared than if they had started seeing patients immediately.

Quick Checklist

Before your first patient, confirm that you have:

□ *Active RN and APRN licenses*

□ *National board certification*

□ *DEA registration (if applicable)*

□ *NPI obtained*

□ *Credentialing initiated or completed*

□ *Malpractice insurance verified*

□ *Employer orientation scheduled*

□ *Access to your electronic health record*

□ *Reliable drug reference resources*

□ *At least one experienced mentor you can contact with questions*

Chapter 2

Imposter Syndrome Is Normal

"Confidence is not a prerequisite for becoming a good clinician. It is the result of practicing thoughtfully, learning continuously, and caring deeply for your patients."

If you have ever thought,
"What if I'm not ready?"
"What if everyone realizes I don't know enough?"
"What if I make the wrong diagnosis?"

You are not alone.

Almost every new PMHNP experiences moments of self-doubt during the transition from student to independent clinician. This feeling has a name: **imposter syndrome**.

Imposter syndrome is the persistent belief that your accomplishments are somehow undeserved and that others will eventually discover you are not as capable as they think. It can affect high-achieving professionals at every stage of their careers, including experienced psychiatrists, psychologists, physicians, nurse practitioners, and educators.

Feeling uncertain does not mean you are unqualified. More often, it means you recognize the responsibility that comes with caring for patients.

Confidence vs. Competence

Many new graduates believe they should feel confident on their first day of practice.

In reality, competence develops before confidence.

Graduate school gave you the knowledge and foundation to begin practicing safely. Your first months—and even years—in practice are where you will develop the clinical judgment that comes only through experience.

Competence grows through repetition, reflection, and continuous learning.

Confidence follows.

Clinical Pearl

Do not confuse uncertainty with incompetence.

The safest clinicians are often the ones who pause, think carefully, and seek guidance when appropriate.

Learning Safely

You are expected to be a competent beginner—not an expert.

Early in your career, focus on developing safe clinical habits.

Take the time to review previous records.

Verify medication histories.

Consult clinical guidelines.

Look up unfamiliar medications.

Discuss challenging cases with experienced colleagues.

Patients benefit when clinicians are thoughtful, not rushed.

Know Your Limits

Every clinician has limitations.

Recognizing them is one of the hallmarks of professionalism.

There will be patients whose presentation is unusually complex.

There will be medications you have prescribed only a few times.

There will be diagnoses that require additional consultation.

Knowing when to seek help protects both your patients and your professional growth.

Common Misstep

Believing you must manage every patient independently simply because you are the treating clinician.

Experienced practitioners routinely consult colleagues, discuss difficult cases, and seek second opinions.

Collaboration is good clinical practice.

Asking for Help

Some new graduates worry that asking questions will make them appear inexperienced.

The opposite is usually true.

Supervisors and experienced clinicians generally appreciate thoughtful questions that demonstrate preparation and critical thinking.

Before seeking consultation:

- Review the patient's chart.
- Organize your thoughts.
- Develop a differential diagnosis.
- Consider an initial treatment plan.

Then ask focused questions.

Rather than saying, *"I don't know what to do,"*
try saying, *"I am considering bipolar II disorder versus recurrent major depressive disorder because of these findings. I would appreciate your thoughts on how you would approach treatment."*
This approach demonstrates clinical reasoning while remaining open to guidance.

Building Confidence

Confidence is not something that suddenly appears after a certain number of patients.

It develops gradually through experience.

You may notice that six months from now, you will recognize patterns that seemed confusing today.

One year from now, you will handle situations that once felt overwhelming.

Growth often happens so gradually that you do not notice it until you look back.

Celebrate those milestones.

Finding Mentors

One of the greatest investments you can make in your career is maintaining relationships with mentors.

Stay connected with:

- Former preceptors
- Collaborating psychiatrists
- Experienced PMHNPs
- Pharmacists
- Therapists
- Primary care colleagues
- Trusted classmates

Mentorship does not end at graduation.

Many of the most meaningful professional opportunities arise from relationships built over time.

Liberty's Lesson

One of the greatest blessings in my career has been the mentors and colleagues who continued to guide me long after I graduated.

I stayed connected with my preceptors, psychiatrists I worked alongside as a registered nurse, former RN colleagues, classmates from nurse practitioner school, and many professionals I met throughout my journey.

Those relationships became sources of wisdom, encouragement, collaboration, and lifelong friendships.

Never underestimate the value of maintaining professional relationships.

Treat people with respect.

Support your colleagues.

Do not burn bridges.

Our profession is smaller than you think, and the relationships you build today may shape opportunities you cannot yet imagine.

Clinical Reasoning in Action

"I Think Everyone Knows More Than I Do"

A newly hired PMHNP finishes her third week in an outpatient clinic. She notices that the psychiatrist next door completes patient visits quickly, makes diagnoses with confidence, and rarely looks anything up.

Meanwhile, she spends extra time reviewing charts, checking medication references, and confirming treatment recommendations before finalizing her notes.

She begins to wonder whether she is falling behind.

During a collaborative meeting, she shares her concerns.

Her collaborating psychiatrist smiles and says,
"You are seeing what I do now. You are not seeing the twenty years it took me to get here."

He explains that he still consults colleagues, reviews new research, and occasionally looks up dosing recommendations.

Experience does not eliminate learning.

It simply changes the kinds of questions you ask.

Quick Checklist

When self-doubt appears, remind yourself:

□ *Competence comes before confidence.*

□ *It is okay to look things up.*

□ *Consultation is a sign of professionalism.*

□ *Every experienced clinician was once a beginner.*

□ *Keep learning, asking questions, and reflecting on your practice.*

□ *Build relationships with mentors who will continue to challenge and support you.*

Clinical Pearl

Your first year is about building a strong foundation—not proving that you already know everything. Every experienced PMHNP once stood exactly where you are today.

Chapter 3

Setting Up Your Clinical Toolkit

"Excellent clinicians are not those who memorize the most information. They are the ones who know where to find reliable information when they need it."

One of the biggest surprises for many new PMHNPs is realizing that experienced clinicians look things up every day.

They consult references.

They review guidelines.

They verify doses.

They compare treatment options.

They read new research.

They ask colleagues for advice.

Clinical excellence is not about having every answer memorized—it is about consistently using trustworthy resources to make safe, evidence-based decisions.

This chapter introduces the tools that should become part of your everyday practice.

Your Core Library

There are a handful of resources that nearly every PMHNP should have readily available. Think of these as the foundation of your professional library.

DSM-5-TR

The **Diagnostic and Statistical Manual of Mental Disorders, Fifth Edition, Text Revision (DSM-5-TR)** remains the primary diagnostic reference for psychiatric practice in the United States.

The DSM-5-TR helps clinicians:

- Apply standardized diagnostic criteria.
- Differentiate psychiatric disorders.
- Improve diagnostic consistency.
- Communicate effectively with other healthcare professionals.
- Support documentation and reimbursement.

Remember that the DSM provides diagnostic criteria—it does **not** replace clinical judgment.

Patients rarely present exactly as described in textbooks.

Clinical Pearl

Use the DSM to organize your thinking—not to replace it.

Psychopharmacology References

Medication management is one of the most dynamic areas of psychiatric practice.
New medications are approved.
Warnings change.
Monitoring recommendations evolve.
Rather than relying on memory alone, become comfortable consulting trusted references before prescribing.

Useful resources include:

- Stahl's Essential Psychopharmacology
- Stahl's Prescriber's Guide
- The Carlat Psychiatry Report
- Maudsley Prescribing Guidelines
- APA Practice Guidelines
- FDA Prescribing Information

Some healthcare insurance websites also have sections for Practice Guidelines.

Experienced clinicians often verify information before prescribing unfamiliar medications.

Drug Information Resources

In addition to textbooks, every PMHNP should have access to current drug databases.

These resources provide:

- Adult dosing
- Geriatric dosing
- Renal adjustments
- Hepatic adjustments
- Drug interactions
- Black Box Warnings
- Pregnancy and lactation information
- Monitoring recommendations

Examples include:

- Lexicomp
- Micromedex
- Epocrates
- Facts & Comparisons

Common Misstep

Prescribing based solely on memory.
Even experienced psychiatrists verify dosing recommendations, medication interactions, and updated prescribing information.
Looking it up protects both you and your patient.

Rating Scales

Rating scales do not replace clinical interviews.
They supplement them.

When used appropriately, they help:

- Establish baseline symptom severity.
- Monitor treatment response.
- Improve documentation.
- Facilitate communication with other providers.

Common examples include:

Rating Scale	Primary Use
PHQ-9	Depression
GAD-7	Anxiety
MDQ	Bipolar Disorder Screening
ASRS	ADHD Screening
PCL-5	PTSD Symptoms
C-SSRS	Suicide Risk Assessment
MMSE	Cognitive Screening
MoCA	Mild Cognitive Impairment
AIMS	Tardive Dyskinesia Monitoring

Use rating scales to inform—not replace—your clinical assessment.

Documentation Templates

Documentation is an essential clinical skill.

Templates can improve efficiency and consistency while ensuring important clinical elements are not overlooked.

Develop templates for:

- Psychiatric evaluations
- Follow-up visits
- Mental Status Examinations
- Suicide risk assessments
- Medication consent discussions
- Controlled substance monitoring

Templates should support thoughtful documentation rather than encourage copy-and-paste notes.

Artificial Intelligence as a Clinical Tool

Artificial intelligence is rapidly changing healthcare.

When used responsibly, AI can improve efficiency, education, and clinical workflow.

Potential uses include:

- Summarizing new research
- Brainstorming differential diagnoses
- Drafting patient education materials
- Creating clinic workflows
- Developing teaching materials
- Generating study guides
- Improving writing and documentation

AI should never replace clinical judgment or independent decision-making.

Always verify information using trusted clinical resources before applying it to patient care.

Never enter protected health information into public AI platforms that are not approved by your organization.

Clinical Pearl

Think of AI as a junior research assistant—not your supervising psychiatrist.

Continuing Education

Graduation is only the beginning.
Excellent clinicians intentionally create a lifelong learning plan.
Consider maintaining a balance between:

- Conferences
- Journal reading
- Podcasts
- Continuing education courses
- Case discussions

- Journal clubs
- Professional organizations

Your goal is not simply to earn continuing education credits.

Your goal is to become a better clinician every year.

Clinical Reasoning in Action

"I Don't Know This Medication"

A new PMHNP evaluates a patient whose medication list includes a recently approved antidepressant that he has never prescribed.
Instead of pretending to be familiar with it, he reviews the prescribing information, consults a trusted drug reference, discusses the medication with his collaborating psychiatrist, and schedules appropriate follow-up before making treatment decisions.

The patient receives safe, evidence-based care.

Professional confidence grows—not because he already knew everything, but because he knew how to find reliable answers.

Liberty's Lesson

One of the greatest lessons I have learned is that no clinician practices alone.

My clinical toolkit extends far beyond books.

It includes mentors I trust, colleagues I respect, pharmacists who willingly answer questions, researchers who challenge my thinking, and students who ask questions that make me reconsider what I thought I knew.

Build your own toolkit intentionally.

Collect resources.

Collect mentors.

Collect experiences.

Over time, they will become just as valuable as your clinical knowledge.

Quick Checklist

Before starting independent practice, make sure you have:

□ *DSM-5-TR*

□ *A trusted psychopharmacology reference*

□ *Drug interaction database*

□ *Rating scales readily available*

□ *Documentation templates*

□ *Reliable AI workflow (HIPAA compliant)*

□ *Access to current clinical guidelines*

□ *A continuing education plan*

□ *Mentors you can contact when needed*

□ *Intellectual curiosity that never stops growing*

Chapter 4

The First Psychiatric Evaluation

"The psychiatric interview is more than a checklist. It is a conversation designed to understand a person's story, identify patterns of illness, assess safety, and develop a treatment plan that fits the individual sitting in front of you."

For many new PMHNPs, the initial psychiatric evaluation feels overwhelming.

There is so much information to gather:

- Why is the patient here?
- What diagnosis fits best?
- Is there a medical cause?
- Are they safe?
- Which medications have already failed?
- What treatment should I recommend?

At first, every evaluation may feel different.

Over time, however, you will discover that experienced clinicians follow a consistent mental framework. The questions change slightly from patient to patient, but the overall structure remains remarkably similar.

The goal of this chapter is to help you develop that structure.

Before You Enter the Room

The psychiatric interview begins **before** you introduce yourself.

Take a few moments to review the chart.

Look for:

- Previous psychiatric diagnoses
- Hospitalizations
- Current medications
- Medication trials
- Allergies
- Medical history
- Recent laboratory studies
- Emergency department visits
- Referral notes
- Previous suicide attempts
- Recent screening questionnaires

This brief preparation helps you ask better questions and identify areas that deserve closer attention.

Clinical Pearl

Never allow the chart to replace the interview.

Use it to guide your questions—not to form conclusions before meeting the patient.

Building Rapport

Patients often decide within the first few minutes whether they trust you.

Introduce yourself clearly.

Explain your role.

Maintain appropriate eye contact.

Allow the patient to tell their story without interruption whenever possible.

Simple phrases such as, *"Tell me what brought you in today."* or *"What concerns you the most?"* often provide more useful information than a series of rapid-fire questions.

Rapport is not simply about being friendly.

It is about creating an environment where patients feel safe enough to share difficult experiences.

The Structure of the Psychiatric Interview

Although every clinician develops their own style, most comprehensive psychiatric evaluations follow a similar sequence.

1. Chief Complaint

Document the patient's primary reason for seeking care, preferably in their own words.

Example: *"I've been anxious for months and can't sleep."*

2. History of Present Illness (HPI)

The HPI is the story of the patient's current illness.

Explore:

- Onset
- Duration
- Severity
- Precipitating factors
- Course over time
- Associated symptoms
- Functional impairment
- Previous treatment
- Current concerns

One helpful strategy is to think chronologically.
How did the symptoms begin?
How have they changed?
What prompted today's visit?

3. Past Psychiatric History

Ask about:

- Previous diagnoses
- Hospitalizations
- Suicide attempts
- Self-injurious behaviors
- Previous medications
- Psychotherapy
- Substance treatment
- Prior psychiatric providers

Past treatment often predicts future treatment response.

4. Medical History
Psychiatry never occurs in isolation.

Many psychiatric symptoms are influenced by medical conditions.

Review:

- Chronic illnesses
- Neurologic disorders
- Endocrine disorders
- Sleep disorders
- Pain conditions
- Surgical history
- Allergies

Remember that depression, anxiety, psychosis, and cognitive impairment may all have medical contributors.

5. Substance Use History

Ask specifically about:

- Alcohol
- Cannabis
- Nicotine
- Opioids
- Stimulants
- Cocaine
- Hallucinogens
- Sedatives
- Energy drinks
- Excessive caffeine

Normalize these questions.
Patients are often more forthcoming when they understand that substance use is a routine part of every psychiatric evaluation.

6. Family Psychiatric History
Family history provides valuable diagnostic clues.

Ask about:

- Depression
- Bipolar disorder
- Schizophrenia
- ADHD
- Autism spectrum disorder
- Substance use disorders
- Suicide

Genetics matter.

7. Social History

One of the most overlooked components of psychiatric care.

Understand the patient's life.

Discuss:

- Childhood
- Education
- Employment
- Military history
- Relationships
- Living situation
- Financial stressors
- Spiritual beliefs
- Legal history
- Trauma exposure
- Social support

Psychiatric symptoms rarely occur in isolation from life circumstances.

8. Mental Status Examination

The Mental Status Examination (MSE) is your psychiatric physical examination.

Observe throughout the interview—not just at the end.

Assess:

- Appearance
- Behavior
- Speech
- Mood
- Affect
- Thought process
- Thought content
- Perception
- Cognition
- Insight
- Judgment

The MSE should reflect what you observed, not what you expected to find.

Time Management

Many new PMHNPs worry that they will not finish the evaluation.

Remember:
The goal is not to ask every possible question.

The goal is to gather enough information to make a safe and thoughtful clinical decision.

If additional information is needed, schedule another visit.

Psychiatric care is a process, not a race.

Common Misstep

Trying to solve every problem during the first visit.

Experienced clinicians prioritize.

Address safety first.

Then diagnosis.

Then treatment.

Everything else can continue over future appointments.

Red Flags That Require Immediate Attention

Certain findings should immediately raise concern:

- Active suicidal intent
- Homicidal intent
- Acute psychosis
- Severe mania
- Delirium
- Catatonia
- Medication toxicity
- Intoxication
- Withdrawal syndromes
- Elder abuse
- Child abuse
- Domestic violence
- Inability to care for basic needs

Recognizing these situations early changes the entire direction of the interview.

Safety always comes first.

Clinical Reasoning in Action

"The Patient Who Wanted ADHD Medication"

A 29-year-old presents requesting stimulant medication for "ADHD."
Rather than immediately focusing on the request, you conduct a complete psychiatric evaluation.

During the interview, you discover episodes of decreased need for sleep, impulsive spending, periods of elevated mood, and a strong family history of bipolar disorder.

Although inattention is present, the broader clinical picture suggests that bipolar disorder should be carefully evaluated before considering stimulant therapy.

The patient's presenting complaint was ADHD.

The patient's actual diagnostic question was much more complex.

Clinical reasoning begins by understanding the whole patient—not simply treating the requested diagnosis.

Liberty's Lesson

One of the most valuable lessons I have learned is this:

Listen longer than feels comfortable.

New clinicians often feel pressure to ask the next question, complete the template, or move through the checklist. But some of the most important clinical information emerges after a brief pause, when the patient realizes they truly have your attention.

Patients do not just come to us for prescriptions—they come to be heard.

Never let documentation become more important than the person sitting in front of you.

Quick Checklist

Before concluding every psychiatric evaluation, ask yourself:

□ *Do I understand why the patient came today?*

□ *Have I ruled out immediate safety concerns?*

□ *Is there a reasonable differential diagnosis?*

□ *Have I considered relevant medical conditions?*

□ *Have I reviewed previous medication trials?*

□ *Do I have enough information to begin treatment safely?*

□ *Does the patient understand the plan?*

□ *Have I arranged appropriate follow-up?*

Chapter 5

Writing Better Notes

"Good documentation is not about writing more. It is about communicating clearly, thinking clinically, and telling the patient's story."

One of the first realities new PMHNPs discover is that documentation occupies a significant portion of the workday. A one-hour psychiatric evaluation may require twenty to thirty minutes—or more—to document thoroughly. Even routine follow-up visits require thoughtful notes that accurately reflect the patient's progress and support the care you provide.

Many clinicians view documentation as paperwork. In reality, documentation is an extension of patient care.

Your note serves several important purposes. It communicates with other healthcare professionals, supports continuity of care, demonstrates medical necessity, justifies treatment decisions, facilitates billing, and provides legal documentation of the encounter. Most importantly, it captures your clinical reasoning.

A well-written note should allow another clinician to answer three questions:

1. *What happened today?*
2. *Why did the clinician make these decisions?*
3. *What happens next?*

If those questions are answered clearly, you have written a good note.

The Four Principles of Excellent Documentation

Every psychiatric note should reflect four essential principles.

1. Be Accurate

Document what you observed, what the patient reported, and what you assessed. Avoid assumptions or conclusions that are not supported by the clinical encounter.

Instead of writing:
Patient is manipulative.

Consider documenting observable behavior:
Patient repeatedly requested early refills despite review of refill policy and became visibly frustrated when alternatives were discussed.

Objective documentation is always stronger than subjective labels.

Clinical Pearl

Describe behaviors—not personalities.

2. Be Concise

More words do not necessarily create a better note.

Include information that contributes to diagnosis, treatment, safety, or continuity of care.

Avoid lengthy narratives that repeat information without adding clinical value.

Experienced clinicians learn to document efficiently without sacrificing quality.

3. Be Clinically Meaningful`

Ask yourself:

Does this information influence today's clinical decision?

Document:

- Symptom severity
- Functional impairment
- Medication response
- Side effects
- Safety concerns
- Patient goals
- Changes since the previous visit

A meaningful note tells the story of the patient's progress—not simply what was discussed.

4. Be Defensible

Every medication change, diagnosis, referral, and follow-up interval should be supported by your clinical reasoning.

Imagine another psychiatrist reviewing your note six months later.

Would they understand why you made your decisions?

If the answer is yes, you have documented well.

Common Misstep

Writing:
"Continue medication."

Instead, explain why:
"Patient reports approximately 60% improvement in depressive symptoms with sertraline 100 mg daily. Denies adverse effects. PHQ-9 decreased from 17 to 8. Will continue current dose and reassess in four weeks."

The second example demonstrates both progress and clinical reasoning.

Tell the Patient's Story

Good psychiatric documentation is more than completing required sections.

It should tell a coherent story.

Imagine your note as a movie rather than a checklist.

The reader should understand:
Who the patient is.

Why they sought treatment.

How they have changed.

What challenges remain.

Why today's treatment plan makes sense.

When documentation tells a clear story, continuity of care improves dramatically.

The Psychiatric Initial Evaluation

A comprehensive psychiatric evaluation generally includes the following sections:

- Chief Complaint
- History of Present Illness
- Past Psychiatric History
- Medical History
- Substance Use History
- Family Psychiatric History
- Social History
- Mental Status Examination
- Risk Assessment
- Assessment and Differential Diagnosis
- Medical Decision Making
- Treatment Plan

Each section should contribute to understanding the patient rather than simply satisfying a documentation requirement.

Writing Better Follow-up Notes

Follow-up documentation should answer one important question:
What has changed since the last visit?

Rather than rewriting the patient's history, focus on:

- Symptom improvement or worsening
- Medication adherence
- Side effects
- Functional changes
- New stressors
- Safety assessment
- Response to treatment

Patients return because their story continues. Your documentation should reflect that progression.

Medical Necessity

Medical necessity is one of the most misunderstood concepts among new clinicians.

Your documentation should explain why today's visit was clinically indicated. Examples include:

- Persistent depressive symptoms requiring medication adjustment
- New adverse effects
- Worsening anxiety affecting work performance
- Monitoring after initiating a controlled substance
- Evaluation of suicidal ideation
- Follow-up after psychiatric hospitalization

When your note explains why care was needed, medical necessity becomes evident.

Risk Assessment

Every psychiatric encounter includes some degree of risk assessment, even if the patient is considered low risk.

Risk documentation should reflect your clinical thinking.

Document:

- Suicidal ideation
- Homicidal ideation
- Self-injurious behavior
- Protective factors
- Access to lethal means (when appropriate)
- Overall acute and chronic risk
- Clinical rationale for disposition

Simply checking "denies SI/HI" is often insufficient.
Explain why outpatient treatment remains appropriate.

Documentation and Artificial Intelligence
Artificial intelligence is beginning to transform clinical documentation.

Used responsibly, AI may assist with:
- Improving grammar
- Organizing note structure
- Drafting patient education materials
- Summarizing literature
- Creating documentation templates

However, AI should never replace independent clinical judgment.

Always verify every statement.

Never enter protected health information into public AI platforms unless they are specifically approved for HIPAA-compliant clinical use.

Clinical Pearl
AI can improve efficiency.
Only you can provide clinical judgment.

Clinical Reasoning in Action
"The Note That Did Not Explain Why"

A PMHNP evaluates a patient with major depressive disorder who reports partial improvement after six weeks of treatment.
The clinician increases the antidepressant dose and schedules follow-up in four weeks.

The original note documents the medication change but does not explain why the dose was increased.

A stronger note might state:
"Patient reports approximately 40% improvement in mood and energy. Continues to experience anhedonia and impaired concentration. Denies adverse effects. Given partial response and good tolerability, will increase escitalopram from 10 mg to 20 mg daily. Risks, benefits, and alternatives discussed. Patient agrees with the plan."

The treatment decision is the same.

The documentation is much stronger.

Liberty's Lesson

One of the most valuable habits I developed was writing notes that I would be comfortable reading years later.

Documentation is not simply a record of what happened. It reflects how you think as a clinician.

As your experience grows, your notes will become shorter, clearer, and more focused—not because you are documenting less, but because you are documenting better.

Always remember that your note may one day be read by another clinician, an auditor, an attorney, or even the patient. Write with professionalism, clarity, and respect.

Quick Checklist

Before signing your note, ask yourself:

□ *Does this note tell the patient's story?*

□ *Have I documented my clinical reasoning?*

□ *Does the note support medical necessity?*

□ *Have I documented risk assessment?*

□ *Have I explained medication changes?*

□ *Is the treatment plan clear?*

□ *Would another clinician understand exactly what happened today?*

Chapter 6

Medication Management

Choosing the Right Medication for the Right Patient

"Prescribing is one of the most powerful tools in psychiatry—but the prescription is only as good as the clinical reasoning behind it."

One of the greatest privileges of becoming a Psychiatric Mental Health Nurse Practitioner is the ability to prescribe medications that can profoundly improve a person's quality of life. The right medication can relieve depression, reduce anxiety, stabilize mood, improve concentration, decrease psychosis, and restore functioning. At the same time, every prescription carries potential risks, adverse effects, interactions, and responsibilities.

New PMHNPs often worry about choosing the "perfect" medication.

In reality, experienced clinicians rarely think in terms of perfect medications. Instead, they ask:
"Which medication is the best fit for this particular patient today?"

Medication management is not simply matching a diagnosis to a drug. It is the thoughtful integration of diagnosis, symptom severity, medical history, previous treatment response, patient preferences, safety considerations, cost, adherence, and long-term goals.

The purpose of this chapter is not to teach every psychiatric medication.
Entire textbooks are dedicated to psychopharmacology. Instead, this chapter teaches **how experienced clinicians approach prescribing**.

Start With the Diagnosis—But Don't Stop There

A diagnosis provides a starting point, not the entire answer.

Two patients may both meet criteria for Major Depressive Disorder but require completely different treatment plans.

One may have:

- severe insomnia
- poor appetite
- weight loss
- anxiety
- financial limitations

Another may have:

- hypersomnia
- obesity
- sexual dysfunction
- ADHD
- hypertension

Although both have the same diagnosis, their medication selection may be very different.

Treat the patient—not just the diagnosis.

Clinical Pearl

Psychiatric medications are prescribed for people, not diagnoses.

Develop a Prescribing Framework

Before writing a prescription, ask yourself several key questions.

What is my working diagnosis?
Be as confident as possible before initiating treatment.

If the diagnosis remains uncertain, consider whether additional history, collateral information, laboratory studies, or follow-up is needed before prescribing.

What symptoms am I treating?
Be specific.

Rather than saying, *"Treat depression,"*
consider:

- depressed mood
- anhedonia
- insomnia
- poor concentration
- panic attacks
- irritability
- impulsivity

Understanding the target symptoms helps you select medications more intentionally and evaluate treatment response over time.

What has already been tried?
One of the most valuable questions you can ask is:
"Tell me about medications you've taken before."

Explore:

- effectiveness
- side effects
- duration
- adherence
- reasons for discontinuation

A medication that failed after two days because of nausea is different from one that was ineffective after an adequate therapeutic trial.

Consider the Whole Patient

Medication selection should always consider factors beyond psychiatric symptoms.

- age
- pregnancy or breastfeeding
- medical conditions
- renal function
- hepatic function
- obesity
- cardiovascular disease
- seizure disorders
- substance use
- financial limitations
- insurance coverage
- ability to adhere to treatment

Every prescription should fit the patient's overall clinical picture.

Shared Decision-Making

Patients are more likely to adhere to treatment when they participate in the decision.

Discuss:

- expected benefits
- common adverse effects
- Black Box Warnings when applicable
- expected timeline for improvement
- alternative treatment options
- risks of declining treatment

Informed consent is an ongoing conversation, not a one-time event.

Start Low, Go Slow—But Know When Not To

Many psychiatric medications should be initiated gradually, particularly in older adults and medically complex patients.

However, "start low and go slow" should not become "start too low and never reach an effective dose."

The goal is thoughtful titration—not unnecessary hesitation.

Monitoring

Prescribing does not end when the prescription is sent.

Follow-up is essential.

Monitor:

- symptom improvement
- side effects
- adherence
- laboratory studies when indicated
- vital signs
- weight
- metabolic parameters
- movement disorders
- patient satisfaction

Treatment is a continuous process of reassessment and adjustment.

When Not to Prescribe

Sometimes the safest prescription is no prescription.

There are situations where delaying medication is appropriate.

Examples include:

- diagnostic uncertainty
- suspected bipolar disorder before antidepressant monotherapy
- intoxication
- medication-seeking behavior
- untreated medical conditions
- patient declines treatment
- need for further evaluation

Resisting pressure to prescribe unnecessarily is an important clinical skill.

Many new PMHNPs feel pressured to prescribe quickly.

Patients may expect to leave with a medication. Employers may emphasize productivity. Even clinicians may feel that every visit should result in a prescription.

Remember that prescribing is only one form of treatment.
Sometimes education, psychotherapy, additional diagnostic clarification, laboratory testing, or close follow-up is the better clinical decision.

Thoughtful restraint is just as important as thoughtful prescribing.

Common Misstep

Prescribing because you feel pressured to "do something."

Every prescription should have a clear indication, expected benefit, monitoring plan, and exit strategy.

Follow-up Intervals

How soon should patients return?

There is no universal answer.

The interval depends on:

- diagnosis
- medication started
- suicide risk
- medication side effects
- patient reliability
- complexity of the case

In general:

- High-risk or newly initiated medications often require earlier follow-up.
- Stable patients may be seen less frequently.

Individualize your plan.

Clinical Reasoning in Action

"The Medication the Patient Requested"

A 34-year-old patient presents requesting alprazolam for anxiety.
Rather than immediately granting or denying the request, you complete a comprehensive evaluation.

The patient reports chronic generalized anxiety, poor sleep, daily cannabis use, and a history of alcohol misuse. Previous records reveal significant improvement on an SSRI that was discontinued after six months because the patient felt better. After discussing treatment options, you recommend restarting the SSRI, initiating cognitive behavioral therapy, improving sleep hygiene, and scheduling close follow-up instead of prescribing a benzodiazepine.

The patient initially appears disappointed but agrees to the plan after understanding the rationale.

The best prescription is not always the one the patient requests.
It is the one most likely to improve long-term health while minimizing harm.

Liberty's Lesson

Early in my career, I thought experienced clinicians succeeded because they always knew the right medication.

Over time, I realized something different.

They succeeded because they consistently asked the right questions before prescribing.

They listened carefully.

They considered alternatives.

They anticipated side effects.

They thought several steps ahead.

Good prescribing begins long before you click "Send" on the prescription.

Quick Checklist

Before prescribing, ask yourself:

□ *Am I confident in the diagnosis?*

□ *What symptom am I treating?*

□ *Have previous medication trials been reviewed?*

□ *Have I considered medical comorbidities?*

□ *Are there potential drug interactions?*

□ *Have I discussed risks, benefits, and alternatives?*

□ *Have I documented informed consent?*

□ *Is there a monitoring plan?*

□ *When should I reassess?*

Chapter 7

Challenging Encounters

Communicating with Confidence, Compassion, and Professional Boundaries

"The most difficult part of psychiatric practice is rarely choosing the right medication. More often, it is navigating difficult conversations while preserving the therapeutic relationship."

Every PMHNP will eventually encounter patients who are angry, frustrated, fearful, demanding, or resistant to treatment.

These encounters can be emotionally draining, especially for new clinicians who worry about saying the wrong thing or damaging rapport.

The good news is that difficult encounters are not signs of failure.
They are a normal part of psychiatric practice.

Patients often come to us during the most stressful periods of their lives. Many have experienced trauma, chronic mental illness, unstable relationships, addiction, grief, or years of feeling misunderstood. Their emotions may emerge during the clinical encounter.

Your role is not to "win" the conversation.
Your role is to remain calm, curious, compassionate, and clinically grounded.

This chapter will help you approach these situations with confidence while maintaining appropriate professional boundaries.

Understand the Behavior Before Reacting to It

One of the most important lessons in psychiatry is this:

Behavior is communication.

A patient's behavior often reflects an unmet need, emotional distress, fear, frustration, or symptoms of illness.
The patient who appears demanding may be anxious.
The patient who becomes angry may feel unheard.
The patient requesting early refills may be struggling with dependence, inadequate symptom control, or both.
Understanding behavior does not mean accepting inappropriate behavior.
It means responding thoughtfully rather than reactively.

Clinical Pearl

Respond to the emotion before responding to the request.
Patients are more likely to hear your recommendations after they feel heard themselves.

When Patients Request Specific Medications

One of the most common situations for new PMHNPs is the patient who arrives with a specific request.
"I need Xanax."
"Adderall is the only thing that works."
"My last provider always gave me this medication."

Avoid immediately agreeing—or immediately refusing.
Instead, become curious.

Ask questions.

Explore the patient's history.

Review previous records when available.

Explain your reasoning clearly and respectfully.
Patients may not always agree with your decision, but they should understand how you arrived at it.

Setting Professional Boundaries

Healthy boundaries protect both the patient and the clinician.

Boundaries include:

- Maintaining appropriate communication channels.
- Following refill policies consistently.
- Starting and ending appointments on time.
- Avoiding dual relationships.
- Being empathetic without becoming personally responsible for solving every problem.

Consistency builds trust.

De-escalating an Angry Patient

When emotions escalate, remember that your demeanor often sets the tone for the encounter.

Practical strategies include:

- Remain calm.
- Lower your voice rather than raising it.
- Avoid interrupting.
- Acknowledge emotions without immediately agreeing with conclusions.
- Set respectful limits when necessary.
- Focus on solutions rather than arguments.

Many conflicts de-escalate simply because the patient feels genuinely heard.

Common Misstep

Trying to prove that you are right.

The goal is not to win an argument.

The goal is to provide safe, compassionate care while maintaining professionalism.

Borderline Personality Disorder: A Shift in Perspective

Patients with borderline personality disorder often evoke strong emotional responses in healthcare providers.

Rather than asking,
"Why is this patient so difficult?"

consider asking,
"What experiences may have shaped this patient's way of relating to others?"

Maintaining consistent boundaries, validating emotions, and avoiding unnecessary power struggles are often more effective than confrontation.

When Family Members Take Over

Family members can provide valuable collateral information, but they can also unintentionally dominate the encounter.

Whenever appropriate, spend part of the visit speaking privately with the patient.

This protects autonomy and may reveal concerns the patient is reluctant to discuss in front of others.

Non-Adherence

Patients stop medications for many reasons.

Sometimes they forget.

Sometimes they cannot afford treatment.

Sometimes adverse effects outweigh benefits.

Sometimes they simply do not believe they need medication.

Approach non-adherence with curiosity rather than judgment.

Understanding the reason is the first step toward improving adherence.

Clinical Reasoning in Action

"The Patient Who Wanted Adderall"

A 27-year-old patient schedules an evaluation stating, "I'm here because I need Adderall."

Rather than immediately discussing stimulants, you complete a comprehensive assessment.

The patient describes lifelong distractibility but also reports nightly cannabis use, untreated anxiety, irregular sleep, and frequent panic attacks.
Instead of framing the visit around a requested medication, you explain that your priority is identifying the underlying cause of the symptoms.

Together, you discuss anxiety management, sleep improvement, and a formal ADHD evaluation before deciding whether stimulant medication is appropriate.

The patient leaves without an Adderall prescription—but with a clear explanation, a collaborative plan, and a follow-up appointment.

Good clinical care begins with understanding the problem, not simply fulfilling the request.

Liberty's Lesson

Some of the most rewarding relationships in psychiatry begin as the most challenging.

Patients may forget the exact medication you prescribed or the dosage you selected, but they often remember how you made them feel during one of the hardest moments of their lives.

Listen carefully.

Speak respectfully.

Hold firm to your clinical judgment.

You can be both compassionate and boundaried.

Those qualities are not opposites—they are the foundation of excellent psychiatric care.

Quick Checklist

Before responding to a challenging situation, ask yourself:

□ *Have I identified the emotion driving the behavior?*

□ *Am I responding calmly rather than reacting emotionally?*

□ *Have I clearly explained my clinical reasoning?*

□ *Have I maintained appropriate professional boundaries?*

□ *Does the patient understand the treatment plan?*

□ *Have I documented the encounter objectively?*

Bonus Feature
Words That Work

A Preview from the Future PMHNP Communication Library

"You do not need the perfect words. You need words that communicate empathy, professionalism, and sound clinical judgment."

1. When a Patient Requests a Controlled Substance

Patient

"I just need Xanax. That's the only thing that works."

Instead of saying…

"I don't prescribe Xanax."

Try…

"I appreciate you sharing what has worked for you in the past. Before we decide on any medication, I'd like to understand your symptoms, treatment history, and goals so we can choose the safest and most effective treatment together."

Why it works:
It acknowledges the patient's experience without committing to the requested medication.

2. When a Patient Becomes Angry
Patient
"You're not listening to me!"

Try…
"I'm sorry it feels that way. I want to make sure I understand what's most important to you today. Tell me what concerns you the most."

Why it works:
It validates emotion without admitting fault and redirects the conversation toward problem-solving.

3. When You Need to Set a Boundary
Patient
"Can't you just refill it this one time?"

Try…
"I understand why you're asking. My responsibility is to provide care that's both compassionate and safe. Let's look at the options that allow us to do both."

Why it works:
It frames the boundary as patient-centered rather than punitive.

4. When the Family Answers Every Question
Try…
"I appreciate your perspective, and it is helpful to hear your observations. I'd also like to spend a few minutes speaking with [the patient] alone, because that's a routine part of every psychiatric evaluation."

Why it works:
It preserves the patient's autonomy while respecting the family's involvement.

5. When You Don't Yet Have the Answer

Patient

"So…what medication are you going to give me?"

Try…

"At this point, I'd like to gather a little more information before making that decision. Sometimes the safest treatment plan begins with a more complete understanding of what's causing the symptoms."

Why it works:

It reinforces that careful evaluation is a strength—not hesitation.

Liberty's Closing Thought

One lesson took me years to fully appreciate:

Patients rarely expect perfection.

They expect honesty.

They appreciate being heard.

They respect clinicians who explain their thinking.

The words you choose can strengthen—or weaken—the therapeutic relationship just as much as the medication you prescribe.

Communication is a clinical skill.

Like every clinical skill, it improves with practice.

Coming in a future volume of the Advanced Practice Series…

The PMHNP Communication Library

Words That Work: Real Conversations in Psychiatric Practice

Practical scripts, difficult conversations, and communication strategies for everyday psychiatric practice.

Chapter 8

Psychiatric Emergencies Every PMHNP Should Recognize

Recognize Early. Respond Appropriately. Protect Your Patient.

"Most psychiatric emergencies are not difficult because they are rare. They are difficult because they require timely recognition, calm clinical judgment, and decisive action."

One of the biggest misconceptions among new PMHNPs is that psychiatric emergencies only occur in emergency departments or inpatient psychiatric units.

The reality is that psychiatric emergencies can present in any setting—outpatient clinics, telepsychiatry visits, primary care offices, nursing facilities, schools, and even routine follow-up appointments.

Fortunately, your responsibility is not to manage every emergency independently.

Your responsibility is to recognize when a patient requires a higher level of care and to respond appropriately.

Recognizing emergencies early often prevents tragedy.

This chapter focuses on identifying red flags, determining when outpatient treatment is no longer appropriate, and coordinating the next level of care.

Think Safety First

Before considering diagnoses or medications, ask yourself one question:
"Is this patient safe to leave today?"

That question should guide every psychiatric encounter.

Safety includes not only suicide and violence risk, but also severe psychosis, impaired judgment, medical instability, intoxication, and the patient's ability to care for themselves.
If the answer is uncertain, pause and reassess before proceeding with routine treatment.

Clinical Pearl

Never allow a busy clinic schedule to rush a safety assessment.

Suicide Risk

Every PMHNP should become comfortable assessing suicide risk.

A suicide assessment is not simply asking,
"Are you suicidal?"

Instead, explore:

- Current suicidal thoughts
- Intent
- Specific plan
- Access to means
- Previous attempts
- Protective factors
- Reasons for living
- Recent stressors
- Substance use
- Impulsivity

Remember that risk exists on a spectrum.

Patients may deny suicidal intent while still requiring close monitoring because of multiple risk factors.

Homicidal Ideation

Although less common, homicidal thoughts require the same thoughtful assessment.

Determine:

- Is there a specific target?
- Is there intent?
- Is there a realistic plan?
- Does the patient have access to weapons?
- Is the threat credible and imminent?

Know your state's legal responsibilities regarding duty to protect or duty to warn.

Documentation should clearly describe your assessment and actions.

Acute Psychosis

Patients experiencing psychosis may present with:

- Command hallucinations
- Severe paranoia
- Delusional thinking
- Disorganized speech
- Marked functional decline
- Poor insight
- Inability to care for themselves

Ask yourself:

Can this patient safely function outside of a supervised setting?

If not, emergency evaluation may be necessary.

Mania

Not every manic patient requires hospitalization.

However, hospitalization should be considered when mania results in:

- Dangerous impulsivity
- Aggression
- Psychosis
- Severe insomnia
- Financial recklessness
- Sexual indiscretion
- Inability to care for basic needs

Severity—not simply diagnosis—determines disposition.

Delirium Is a Medical Emergency

One of the easiest mistakes for new clinicians is confusing delirium with a primary psychiatric illness.

Features suggesting delirium include:

- Sudden onset
- Fluctuating level of consciousness
- Disorientation
- Visual hallucinations
- Medical illness
- Infection
- Medication change

Always think medically before assuming psychiatric disease.

Common Misstep

Assuming new confusion in an older adult is dementia or depression.

Acute cognitive change should always prompt evaluation for delirium until proven otherwise.

Medication Emergencies

Although uncommon, every PMHNP should recognize conditions that require immediate medical evaluation.

These include:

- Neuroleptic Malignant Syndrome (NMS)
- Serotonin Syndrome
- Severe lithium toxicity
- Valproate toxicity
- Severe allergic reactions
- Stevens-Johnson Syndrome
- Clozapine-related agranulocytosis or myocarditis (when suspected)

You do not need to diagnose these conditions with certainty.

You need to recognize the warning signs and act promptly.

Intoxication and Withdrawal

Substance-related emergencies may resemble psychiatric illness.

Consider intoxication or withdrawal when patients present with:

- Agitation
- Hallucinations
- Tremors
- Confusion
- Seizures
- Autonomic instability
- Marked behavioral changes

A careful substance use history can dramatically change your differential diagnosis.

Telepsychiatry Emergencies

Psychiatric emergencies during telehealth require additional preparation.

Before beginning a telehealth visit, know:

- The patient's physical location
- A reliable phone number
- An emergency contact
- The nearest emergency department, if feasible

If an emergency arises, remain connected while arranging emergency services whenever possible.

Preparation before the visit often determines how smoothly an emergency can be managed.

When Should You Send the Patient to the Emergency Department?

Emergency evaluation should be considered when patients present with:

- Imminent suicide risk
- Imminent violence risk
- Acute psychosis with inability to remain safe
- Severe mania with impaired judgment
- Delirium
- Medication toxicity
- Catatonia

- Inability to care for basic needs
- Significant medical instability

When in doubt, err on the side of patient safety.

Clinical Reasoning in Action

"Something Didn't Feel Right"

A 72-year-old patient presents for follow-up with increasing confusion, visual hallucinations, and agitation that began two days ago.
The family wonders whether this is "the dementia getting worse."

Instead of immediately adjusting psychiatric medications, you recognize the acute onset and fluctuating symptoms. The patient is referred to the emergency department, where evaluation reveals a urinary tract infection with delirium.

The psychiatric symptoms improve significantly after treatment of the underlying medical condition.

Not every behavioral change is psychiatric.

Sometimes the most important psychiatric decision is recognizing a medical emergency.

Liberty's Lesson

One of the most reassuring realizations in my career was understanding that I didn't need to manage every emergency by myself.

I needed to recognize when the situation exceeded what could safely be managed in the outpatient setting.

Knowing when to escalate care is not a weakness.

It is sound clinical judgment.
Patients are safest when clinicians understand both the strengths and the limits of outpatient psychiatric practice.

Quick Checklist

Before the patient leaves, ask yourself:

□ *Is the patient safe today?*

□ *Have I assessed suicide and violence risk?*

□ *Could this presentation have a medical cause?*

□ *Is outpatient treatment still appropriate?*

□ *Have I documented my clinical reasoning?*

□ *Does the patient understand the next steps?*

□ *Does someone need to be notified or involved in the plan?*

Chapter 9

Clinical Formulation: Turning Information into Insight

A diagnosis tells you what the patient has. A formulation helps you understand why.

"Excellent psychiatric care begins long before the prescription is written. It begins by making sense of the patient's story."

One of the most significant transitions you will make as a new PMHNP is learning that psychiatric practice is not simply about assigning diagnoses.

Graduate school teaches diagnostic criteria.
Clinical practice teaches formulation.

Two patients may both meet DSM-5-TR criteria for Major Depressive Disorder yet require remarkably different treatment plans because the factors contributing to their illness are entirely different.

One patient may be grieving.

Another may have untreated sleep apnea.

A third may be trapped in an abusive relationship.

A fourth may have bipolar disorder presenting as depression.

The diagnosis may be the same.
The formulation is different.

Learning to formulate rather than simply diagnose is what separates competent clinicians from exceptional ones.

What Is Clinical Formulation?

Clinical formulation is your explanation of **why this patient is experiencing these symptoms at this particular time.**

Rather than organizing information into isolated categories, formulation brings the entire story together.

It answers questions such as:

Why now?

What contributed to this illness?

What continues to maintain it?

What strengths can be used during recovery?

Which interventions are most likely to succeed?

Think of formulation as connecting the dots.

Without it, your note becomes a collection of facts.

With it, the facts become a coherent clinical story.

Looking Beyond the Diagnosis

The DSM provides a common language for diagnosis.

That language is essential.

However, diagnoses alone rarely explain the complexity of psychiatric illness.

Consider two patients diagnosed with generalized anxiety disorder.

One developed anxiety after surviving a traumatic event.

The other has lifelong anxiety associated with perfectionism and family history.

Although both meet diagnostic criteria, their treatment plans will likely differ.

Clinical formulation reminds us that people are not diagnoses.

They are individuals whose biology, psychology, relationships, environment, and lived experiences all influence their mental health.

The Five Ps of Clinical Formulation

Many clinicians organize their thinking using the **Five Ps**.

Predisposing Factors

These are the vulnerabilities that increase the likelihood of developing illness.

Examples include:

- Family history
- Genetics
- Early childhood adversity
- Temperament
- Neurodevelopmental conditions
- Chronic medical illness

These factors existed before the current episode.

Precipitating Factors

These are the events that triggered the current symptoms.

Examples include:

- Relationship loss
- Bereavement
- Job loss
- Medical illness
- Substance use
- Academic stress
- Financial difficulties

These answer the question:
Why now?

Perpetuating Factors

These are the factors that keep the illness going.

Examples include:

- Poor sleep
- Avoidance behaviors
- Rumination
- Ongoing substance use
- Family conflict
- Medication nonadherence
- Social isolation

Unless perpetuating factors are addressed, improvement may be limited despite appropriate medications.

Protective Factors

Psychiatry should never focus only on problems.
Protective factors often determine resilience.

Examples include:

- Supportive family
- Insight
- Employment
- Spiritual beliefs
- Stable housing
- Motivation for treatment
- Healthy coping skills

These become valuable assets during recovery.

Presenting Problems

Finally, summarize what brought the patient to treatment.

Include:

- Symptoms
- Functional impairment
- Patient goals
- Immediate concerns

This keeps the formulation connected to the patient's lived experience rather than becoming an academic exercise.

Building a Treatment Plan from the Formulation

Once your formulation is complete, the treatment plan often becomes much clearer.

For example:
If insomnia perpetuates depression…
Treat sleep.

If alcohol worsens anxiety…
Address alcohol use.

If social isolation maintains symptoms…
Encourage meaningful social engagement.

If trauma drives emotional dysregulation…
Trauma-informed psychotherapy becomes essential.

Medication may still be appropriate.
But medication becomes one part of a broader strategy rather than the entire treatment plan.

Common Mistakes

New clinicians often make predictable formulation errors.

One is focusing exclusively on symptoms while overlooking contributing factors.

Another is assuming that the first diagnosis explains every symptom.

A third is failing to identify strengths and protective factors.

Remember that formulation should answer:
"What makes sense about this patient's presentation?"
rather than simply, *"Which diagnosis fits best?"*

Common Misstep

Writing an assessment that simply repeats the diagnosis.

A strong assessment explains **why** you reached your conclusions and how that reasoning guides your treatment plan.

Clinical Formulation Evolves

A formulation is never permanent.

As you learn more about your patient, your understanding changes.

The patient initially diagnosed with major depression may later reveal a history of hypomania.

The patient thought to have ADHD may instead have untreated anxiety and chronic sleep deprivation.

The patient with recurrent panic attacks may ultimately have hyperthyroidism.

Good clinicians update their formulation as new information emerges.

Changing your formulation is not inconsistency.

It is good clinical practice.

Clinical Reasoning in Action

The Patient Who Wasn't "Just Depressed"

A 36-year-old teacher presents with fatigue, poor concentration, insomnia, and loss of interest after several months of declining performance at work.

At first glance, she meets criteria for Major Depressive Disorder.

As you continue the interview, you learn that she recently became the primary caregiver for her father with dementia, sleeps only four to five hours each night, has stopped exercising, and worries constantly about finances.

Rather than viewing her depression as an isolated disorder, your formulation recognizes multiple interacting contributors: caregiver stress, chronic sleep deprivation, anxiety, social withdrawal, and diminished self-care.
Your treatment plan reflects this broader understanding. Along with discussing antidepressant therapy, you explore caregiver support resources, recommend psychotherapy, address sleep hygiene, and help her identify realistic ways to restore self-care.

The diagnosis explains **what** she has.

The formulation explains **why** she is struggling—and points toward a more comprehensive treatment plan.

Liberty's Lesson

One of the greatest compliments you can receive from a patient is:
"You really understand what's been happening to me."

That statement rarely comes from naming the correct diagnosis.
It comes from understanding the whole person.

Every symptom has a context.

Every behavior has a story.

Every patient deserves more than a label.

When you learn to see patterns instead of isolated problems, psychiatry becomes less about treating disorders and more about helping people reclaim their lives.

Quick Checklist

Before finalizing your assessment, ask yourself:

□ *Have I explained* **why** *the patient is experiencing symptoms now?*

□ *Have I identified predisposing, precipitating, perpetuating, and protective factors?*

□ *Does my treatment plan logically follow from my formulation?*

□ *Have I recognized the patient's strengths as well as their challenges?*

□ *Could new information change my current understanding?*

Chapter 10

Protecting Your License

Good Clinical Judgment Is Your Best Risk Management Strategy.

"Your license is one of the most valuable assets you will ever own. Protecting it is not about practicing fearfully—it's about practicing thoughtfully."

Many new PMHNPs worry about lawsuits, board complaints, or malpractice claims.

Ironically, the clinicians who worry the most are often the ones least likely to experience serious professional problems.

The greatest risk usually comes from becoming rushed, complacent, or inconsistent.

Most disciplinary actions do not occur because a clinician made one unavoidable mistake.

They occur because small lapses gradually become routine.

Protecting your license begins with the habits you develop every day.

Think Like a Professional Every Day

Every patient encounter should answer three questions:
Was my evaluation thorough?
Was my treatment reasonable?
Can my documentation explain my thinking?

If the answer to all three is yes, you have already reduced much of your professional risk.

Remember:
Your documentation is not simply a record of what happened.
It is evidence of how you thought.

Clinical Pearl

If another clinician reads your note six months from now, they should understand exactly why you made your decisions.

Documentation Is Your Strongest Defense

Good documentation protects:

- Your patient
- The next clinician
- Continuity of care
- Medical necessity
- Your professional judgment

Avoid documenting only conclusions.
Instead, document your reasoning.

Rather than writing:
"Low suicide risk."

Explain why.
For example:
The patient denies suicidal ideation, has no history of attempts, demonstrates future-oriented thinking, identifies strong family support, and agrees to seek emergency care if symptoms worsen.

Reasoning carries far more value than labels.

Controlled Substances Require Consistency

Prescribing controlled medications is part of psychiatric practice, but it requires clear boundaries.

Develop office policies that are applied consistently.

Consider documenting:

- Diagnosis supporting treatment
- Review of previous records

- PDMP review when required
- Risks and benefits discussed
- Follow-up plan
- Refill expectations

Consistency protects both the patient and the clinician.

Common Misstep

Making exceptions "just this once."
One inconsistent decision often becomes difficult to explain later.

Professional Boundaries Matter

Patients may ask for favors that seem harmless:

- Personal phone numbers
- Social media connections
- Letters that stretch beyond your clinical findings
- Medication refills without evaluation
- Informal advice outside scheduled visits

Maintaining boundaries does not weaken rapport.
It strengthens trust.

Patients deserve consistency, fairness, and professionalism.

Telepsychiatry Responsibilities

Virtual care carries the same professional responsibilities as in-person practice.

Before each visit:

- Confirm patient identity.
- Verify the patient's physical location.
- Ensure privacy.
- Have emergency contact information available.
- Know local emergency resources when possible.

The standard of care remains the same regardless of the setting.

Mandatory Reporting

Every PMHNP should understand the reporting requirements in the state where they practice.

Examples may include:

- Suspected child abuse
- Elder abuse
- Dependent adult abuse
- Certain threats of violence
- Other state-specific legal obligations

Know the laws before you need them.

When uncertain, consult your organization's policies, supervisor, legal counsel, or licensing board guidance.

Receiving a Complaint

Sooner or later, nearly every experienced clinician encounters an unhappy patient.

A complaint does not necessarily mean you provided poor care.

Remain professional.

Avoid defensive communication.

Review the record carefully.

Seek guidance from your malpractice carrier or employer when appropriate.

Most concerns are resolved through thoughtful communication and complete documentation.

Your Reputation Is Built One Encounter at a Time

Professionalism extends beyond the examination room.

It includes:

- Respectful communication
- Timely documentation
- Reliable follow-up
- Collegial collaboration
- Honest acknowledgment of mistakes
- Lifelong learning

Your reputation often becomes your greatest professional asset.

Protect it as carefully as you protect your license.

Clinical Reasoning in Action

"The Missed Refill Request"

A patient sends multiple portal messages requesting an early refill of a controlled medication late on Friday afternoon.

Rather than automatically approving the request or declining without explanation, you review the chart, check the prescription monitoring program as required, and compare the refill history with the treatment agreement.

You discover repeated early refill requests over several months that had not previously been addressed.

Instead of continuing the pattern, you document your review, explain your concerns to the patient, schedule an earlier follow-up visit, and discuss safer long-term management.

The issue was not the refill itself.

It was recognizing a pattern that required clinical attention.

Liberty's Lesson

Throughout this book, we've talked about confidence.

Many new PMHNPs believe confidence comes from knowing every diagnosis or every medication.

In my experience, confidence comes from something different.

It comes from practicing with integrity.

It comes from being willing to ask questions, document your reasoning, admit uncertainty, continue learning, and place the patient's well-being at the center of every decision.

If you build those habits early, your confidence will grow naturally.
And so will the trust your patients place in you.

Quick Checklist

Before ending each clinic day, ask yourself:

□ *Are today's notes complete?*

□ *Did I document my clinical reasoning?*

□ *Did I address safety concerns?*

□ *Were controlled substances prescribed consistently?*

□ *Have I maintained professional boundaries?*

□ *Are follow-up plans clearly documented?*

□ *If another clinician reviewed today's charts tomorrow, would my decisions make sense?*

EPILOGUE

When you began this journey, you were preparing to become a PMHNP. Today, you have a practical framework for evaluating patients, documenting thoughtfully, prescribing safely, navigating difficult encounters, recognizing emergencies, formulating cases, and protecting your professional practice. You will continue learning throughout your career—but you are no longer beginning. You are building the habits of a thoughtful psychiatric clinician.

www.ingramcontent.com/pod-product-compliance
Lightning Source LLC
LaVergne TN
LVHW010737061126
851857LV00014B/1529